Save Your Kidneys

by

Philip J. Tuso, M.D.

Bloomington, IN 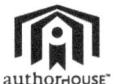 Milton Keynes, UK

authorHOUSE™

AuthorHouse™
1663 Liberty Drive, Suite 200
Bloomington, IN 47403
www.authorhouse.com
Phone: 1-800-839-8640

AuthorHouse™ UK Ltd.
500 Avebury Boulevard
Central Milton Keynes, MK9 2BE
www.authorhouse.co.uk
Phone: 08001974150

First published by AuthorHouse   1/26/2007

ISBN:142593045X(sc)

Library of Congress Control Number: 2006903108

Printed in the United States of America
Bloomington, Indiana

This book is printed on acid-free paper.

Disclaimer

This book was written to help individuals with kidney disease and those who are at risk for developing kidney disease, understand how to save their kidneys. The creator of this book does not warrant or assume any legal liability or responsibility for the accuracy, completeness, or usefulness of any information contained in this book.

The author of this book does not endorse or recommend any commercial products, processes, or services mentioned in this book. The views and opinions of the author expressed in this book do not necessarily state or reflect those of your health care professional team, kidney specialist, or your primary care physician.

It is not the intention of the author of this book to provide specific medical advice but rather to provide users with information about kidney disease. Specific medical advice is not being provided. The author urges you to consult with a qualified physician for diagnosis and answers to your personal questions.

Table of Contents

I. Introduction   1

II. Know Kidney Disease   4

   What is a kidney?   4
   What is kidney disease or renal failure? 6
   What causes kidney disease?   7
   How do we diagnose kidney disease?   8
   What are the signs of kidney disease?   9
   What do kidneys do?   10
   Do you have kidney disease?   12
   How can we save our kidneys?   13
   Kidney disease assessment   14
   Blood testing and treatment quiz   15
   Kidney disease management quiz   16
   Measurable outcomes and goals   17

III. Save Your Kidneys   19

   Kidney function and kidney stage   19
   Why is kidney therapy so important?   24
   Reduce the pressure inside the kidneys   28
   Reduce the pressure outside the kidney   32
   Prevent damage inside the kidney   38

IV. Complications of Kidney Disease   44

   Prevent malnutrition   44
   Prevent anemia   49
   Prevent bone disease   50
   Prevent hyperkalemia   53
   Prevent Hepatitis B infections   55

V. Kidney Replacement Therapy   56

    Hemodialysis   57
    Peritoneal Dialysis   60
    Transplantation   62
    No treatment   65

VI. Conclusion   66

VII. References   67

VIII. Resources   68

I. Introduction

There are two types of kidneys in the world: the "saved kidney" and the "unsaved kidney." The saved kidney is clean and healthy. The unsaved kidney is darkened and diseased.

On the cover of the books are three circles in which the words "Save Your Kidneys" are enclosed. Each circle represents a cross section of a blood vessel inside your kidney. When blood vessels get diseased they cause the lumen (or inside portion) of the blood vessel to occlude (close up) as shown below.

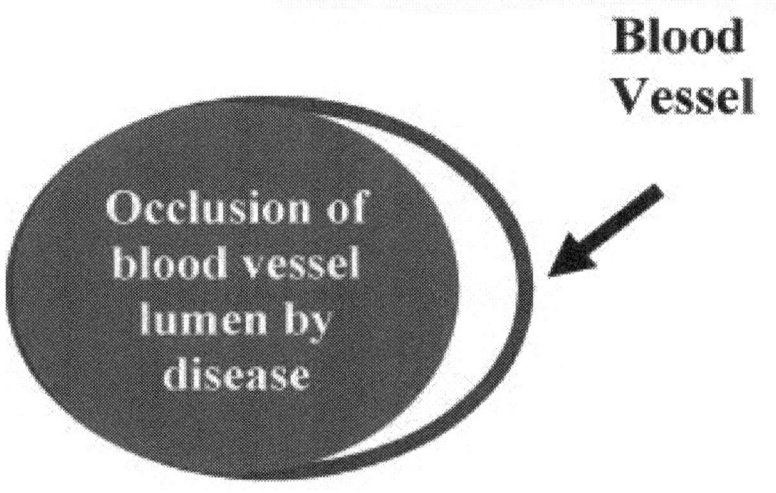

Blood Vessel

Occlusion of blood vessel lumen by disease

Occluded or diseased blood vessels are usually unsaved and will result in unsaved kidneys and kidney failure. The goal of the "Save Your Kidneys" program is to take saved kidneys and prevent them from becoming unsaved. When we start to treat kidney disease, we initiate a plan to prevent further blood vessel injury or further blood vessel occlusion. As a result, the kidney remains healthy and lives longer. We prevent the saved kidney from becoming an unsaved kidney.

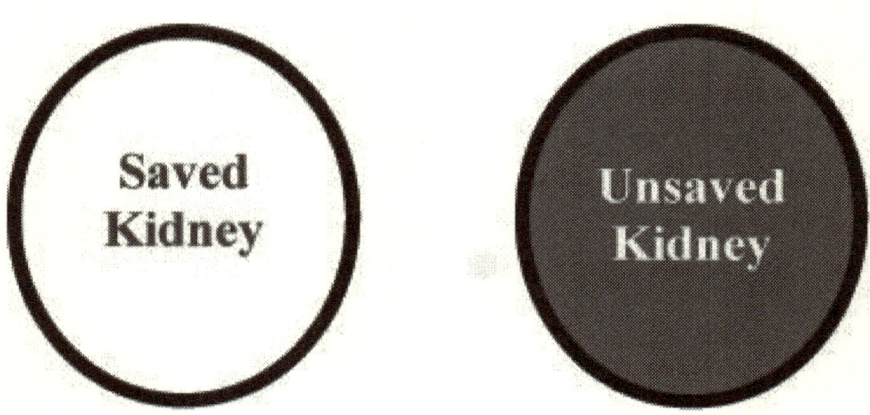

Everyone reading this book is at risk for developing kidney disease sometime in their life. Preventing vascular disease and occlusion of blood vessels is the most effective treatment and prevention of kidney disease. It is also the most effective treatment and prevention of heart disease, strokes, high blood pressure, and diabetes.

Even though I called this book "Save Your Kidneys", the lessons learned in this book can be used to "Save Your Heart" (prevent heart attack), "Save Your Brain (prevent stroke), and Save Your Life." It is pretty much all about the plumbing. Our goal is to keep all blood vessels open and thriving.

This goal can be reached using a simple process that we will teach you in this book.

- Know your numbers
- Know your health care goals
- Determine your plan to achieve your goals
- Write your goals down
- Review on a regular basis

Additional Advice

- Adjust your strategy and goals as needed
- Talk to your health care provider if you have trouble meeting your goals
- Set a new goal when the present one is attained
- Have a positive attitude and have fun

II. Know Kidney Disease

What is a kidney?

The first obvious question is "what is a kidney?" We are born with two kidneys and they are located in the middle of your back on either side of the spine. Each kidney is about the size of your fist. The basic excretory unit of the human kidney is called the nephron. A human kidney contains millions of nephrons. Blood that needs to be cleaned enters the kidneys through the renal artery. After blood is cleaned by the millions of tiny nephrons in your kidneys, it returns to the body through the renal vein. Excess water and waste products are excreted into the urine. Urine is excreted from the kidney into a very thin tube called the ureter. Each kidney connects to a single ureter that takes the urine to the bladder where urine is stored until we go to the bathroom. The urine is removed from the body through the urethra.

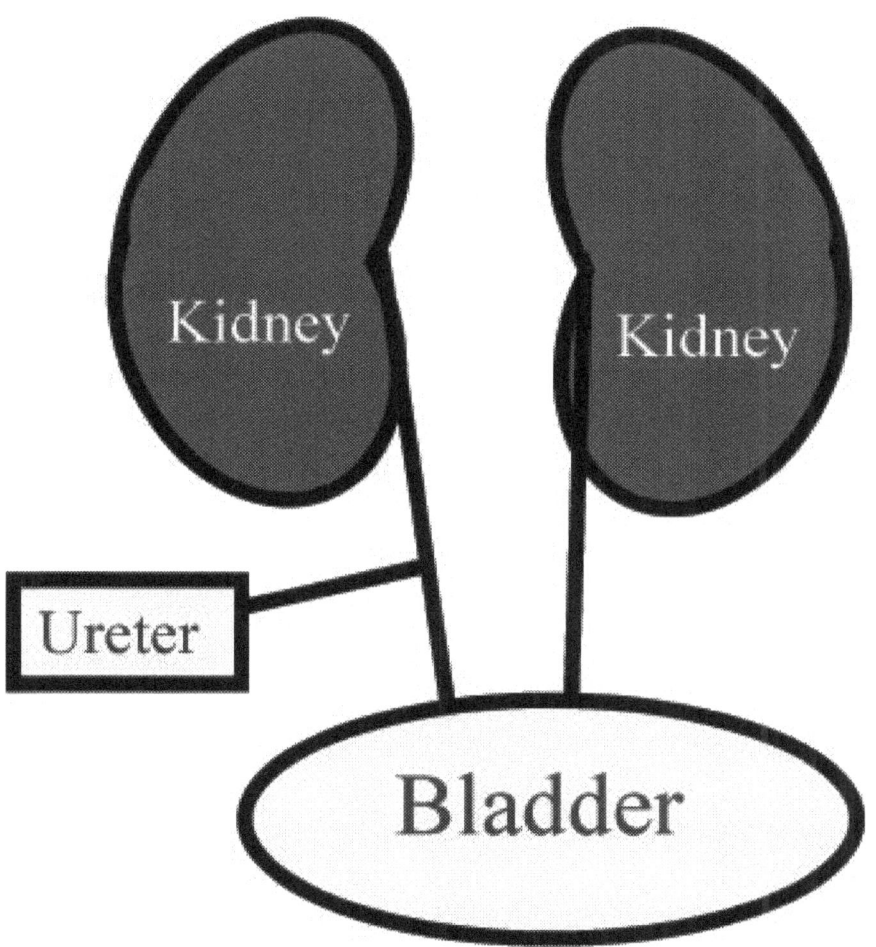

What is kidney disease or renal failure?

Kidney Disease and Renal Failure is the loss of the kidneys ability to adequately perform critical functions, such as excretion of wastes and excretion of water. Most kidney diseases destroy both kidneys simultaneously and the damage can occur slowly over many years. The process is usually painless. Most people with kidney disease do not even know they have kidney disease. Gradual loss of kidney function is commonly referred to as chronic kidney disease or CKD. Persons with chronic kidney disease may go on to develop permanent kidney failure. The condition of total permanent kidney failure is called End Stage Renal Disease (ESRD). Persons with ESRD must undergo dialysis or transplantation to stay alive.

What causes kidney disease?

In the United States, about 20 million Americans have Chronic Kidney Disease (CKD). The most common causes of CKD are diabetes mellitus and high blood pressure. Less common causes of CKD include glomerulonephritis (inflammation of the kidneys), polycystic kidney disease (many cysts inside and outside the kidney) and obstruction of the tubes that send urine from the kidney to the bladder. Common causes of obstruction include kidney stones and cancer. The mortality rate for severe kidney disease can be as high as the mortality rate for renal failure. This means at the end of a five year period one out of two individuals with kidney failure will die.

How do we diagnose kidney disease?

The diagnosis of kidney disease can be made using three simple tests. These include a urine test for protein or albumin (proteinuria), calculation of percent of kidney function from a blood test, and an ultrasound imaging study of the kidneys. Patients with kidney failure usually have protein in the urine, lab tests showing low percent of kidney function and small kidneys by ultrasound (less than 10 centimeters in length). For some patients, simple tests cannot make a diagnosis of kidney disease and the caring physician may recommend a kidney biopsy to confirm the cause of kidney disease. After kidney disease is diagnosed, the patient is usually referred to a kidney specialist or a nephrologist. The nephrologist will help manage complications of kidney disease which may include uremia (accumulation of excess waste products in the body), anemia (low blood counts) and bone disease.

What are the signs of kidney disease?

The signs and symptoms of a person with kidney failure may include increased or decreased urination, fatigue, itching, loss of appetite, unintentional weight loss, nausea and vomiting, swelling or numbness, drowsiness, difficulty concentrating, increased blood pressure, darkening of the skin, muscle cramps, headache, bleeding or bruising easily and frequent hiccups.

What do kidneys do?

When the kidneys no longer do their job, water and waste products accumulate in our body. If we are unable to eliminate water from our body we start to swell. Swelling can occur first in the face around the eyes and eventually in our legs. This is called edema. Increased water in our body can eventually put pressure on our heart and fluid can leak back into our lungs. This results in shortness of breath and may raise our blood pressure.

Urea is a breakdown product of protein that is removed from the body by excretion into the urine. Urea is toxic to our body and needs to be removed daily. When urea accumulates in the body of someone with kidney failure they may lose their appetite and complain of headaches and being tired all the time. In severe cases, kidney failure will cause confusion and even sudden death. Forty years ago, we had no treatment for kidney failure. Today, kidney failure is treated by dialysis or transplantation.

Our kidneys perform many important functions. First, they remove excess fluid from our body. When we drink fluids, our kidneys determine how much fluid we need in our body to stay healthy and what needs to be eliminated. Excess fluid is eliminated in the urine. The other vital function of the kidney is the elimination of salt. A high salt diet can raise our blood pressure and make us feel bloated from fluid retention. When we eat a salty meal, the kidney controls how much salt we need in our body and how much salt needs to be excreted in the urine. In kidney failure, our bodies cannot get rid of salt and our blood pressure will increase even if we eat a low salt diet.

As stated above, the kidney removes toxins or waste products produced by the digestion of food and the rebuilding of our muscles, bones and other vital organs. The waste products are eliminated from our body in our stool and urine.

The kidney also produces two hormones that are important in keeping our bones strong and making sure we have enough red blood cells to circulate oxygen throughout our bodies. The kidney produces the active form of Vitamin D. Vitamin D is generated in our skin by sun exposure. Vitamin D can also be absorbed from our intestinal tract from our diet. Vitamin D requires activation before it helps us absorb mineral that keeps our bones strong. Activation of Vitamin D occurs first in the liver and then in the kidneys. When our liver or our kidneys fail, we cannot produce active Vitamin D and our bones gradually start to break down.

The kidneys also make a hormone called erythropoietin or EPO. This hormone tells the bone marrow to make more red blood cells when our red blood cells get old and die. Without EPO we become anemic and may feel tired and complain of no energy.

Do you have kidney disease?

We know we have kidney disease from blood and urine tests. The severity of kidney disease can be determined by calculating our kidney function and compare it to normal kidney function for our age. Using this concept, we can divide kidney disease into different stages such as mild, moderate, severe kidney disease and kidney failure. An individual with kidney disease should know the percent their kidney is functioning normally. This information helps that patient and the caring physician develop a treatment plan. Obviously there is more urgency to develop a treatment plan if the kidney function is 30% as opposed to 80%. In addition, your physician may advise you on a specific diet and medications that will be started as kidney function deteriorates to less then 30%. When kidney function goes below 20% it is time to prepare mentally and physically for renal replacement therapy.

How can we save our kidneys?

The focus of this book is to "Save Your Kidneys," and show you how to slow down or even prevent kidney disease. People with kidney disease should be pro-active, and develop a plan to save remaining kidney function so they can delay onset and treatment of kidney failure. For example, if someone has 50% kidney function and does nothing to help their kidneys, they may lose 10% kidney function per year and may need dialysis in four years. However, if the same individual can develop a treatment plan that helps prevent kidney injury, they may lose only 5% of their kidney function per year and my not need dialysis for 8-10 years. If kidney function loss can be slowed down to 1% per year, the patient may never need dialysis.

The kidneys are vascular organs that receive blood from the heart. The blood vessels of the body can be compared to the plumbing system in our homes. As the pipes in your home get clogged with dirt, hair and rust, the flow of water through the pipes gets disrupted. This may result in a decrease in water pressure or even a leak that requires re-piping. Diseases like diabetes mellitus, high blood pressure, high cholesterol, obesity and injury from tobacco products affect our bodies plumbing system causing blood vessels to get clogged and injured. Over time, if these diseases are not treated, the blood vessels going to our vital organs (brain, heart, and kidneys) get occluded and damage the organ they are supplying blood to. Therefore, to protect our kidney from damage and to prevent further loss of kidney function we must control blood pressure, control blood sugar (if you have diabetes mellitus), avoid obesity, control blood cholesterol, avoid kidney toxins, and stop smoking.

Kidney disease assessment

Before we get started on your road to renal protection, let us do two short self-assessment tests of your knowledge of what studies should be performed annually to assess your kidney function and if you have an understanding of your kidney health care goals. For each test, give yourself one point for a "yes" answer and no points for a "no" answer. You may also check the box for all "yes" answers and leave the box blank for all "no" answers. When finished, add up all your "yes" answers and determine if you are doing all that you can to prevent and treat kidney disease.

Blood testing and treatment quiz

❏ Do you know your stage of kidney disease?

❏ Have you had a blood test performed for kidney function in the last year?

❏ Have you had a urine test for protein in the last year?

❏ Has your blood pressure been checked in the last year?

❏ Are you taking a blood pressure medication that reduces the pressure inside your kidneys?

❏ Are you taking blood pressure medication that decreases the pressure outside your kidneys?

❏ Have you had blood tests to determine your serum creatinine in the last year?

❏ Have you had a blood test performed for serum cholesterol in the last year?

❏ Have you had your blood tested for diabetes in the last year?

❏ Have you been given a list of medications that are harmful to your kidneys?

If your score is 8-10 you are getting adequate testing and treatment for kidney disease.

If your score is 7 or less than you have an opportunity to improve your kidney care.

Kidney disease management quiz

- ❑ Is your blood pressure less than 130/80 mmHg?
- ❑ Is your blood hematocrit level greater than 30 percent?
- ❑ Is your serum albumin level greater than 3.5 grams per deciliter
- ❑ Is your serum potassium level less than 5.5 milli-equivalents per liter?
- ❑ Is your serum calcium level between 8.4 to 9.5 milligrams per deciliter?
- ❑ Is your serum phosphorus level less than 5.5 milligrams per deciliter?
- ❑ Is your parathyroid hormone level less than 180 pico-grams per milliliter
- ❑ Is your serum low density lipoprotein (LDL) less than 100 milligrams per deciliter?
- ❑ If you have diabetes, is your HgbA1C level less than 6.5%?
- ❑ Is your Hepatitis B surface antibody positive?

If your score is 8-10 you are meeting most of your management goals and are optimizing your ability to slow down kidney disease progression.

If your score is 7 or less than you are not meeting your management goals and are increasing your risk for developing kidney failure and the need to start dialysis therapy.

Measurable outcomes and goals

The kidney is truly an amazing organ that keeps our body in balance. Without a good long term strategy, you run the risk of dying from complications of vascular disease and kidney failure. When kidneys are diseased, your electrolytes and hormones will get out of balance. Blood tests are performed to make sure your kidneys are working properly.

Your doctor will give you a treatment plan and should give you copy of your lab test results. If not, you should ask your doctor for your test results. All tests results should be kept in a folder or notebook for easy reference. When you get your laboratory test results make sure all the tests needed to assess your kidney function have been performed. A sample of a basic chart showing your measurable outcomes and goals is included in this section and at the back of the book for your review. Understanding your goals and plan to achieve these goals is one of the main purposes of this book.

Outcome Measure	Goal
Kidney Function	Greater than 90%
- Creatinine	0.6 to 1.1 mg/dL
- Urine protein	Negative
High Potassium	
- Serum Potassium	3.5 - 5.0 meq/liter
Acidosis	
- Serum Bicarbonate	21 – 31 meq/liter
Bone Disease	
- Calcium	8.5 - 10.5 mg/dL
- Phosphorus	2.7 - 4.5 mg/dL
- PTH	60 - 180 pg/mL
Anemia	
- Hemoglobin	12 - 16 g/dL
Protein Nutrition	
- Albumin	3.5 – 4.8 g/dL
Blood Vessel Disease	
- LDL	Less than 100 mg/dL
- HgbA1C (diabetes)	4.2 - 6.7 %
- Systolic Blood Pressure	Less than 130 mmHg
- Tobacco Use	No
Vaccinations	
- Hepatitis B Antibody	Positive
- Pneumonia	Positive

III. Save Your Kidneys

Kidney function and kidney stage

The definition of Chronic Kidney Disease (CKD) is kidney damage for greater than three months or kidney function testing which shows that the kidney is working less than 60 percent of normal. The percent kidney function tells you what percent your kidney is functioning in the normal range. It is calculated using a computer program that takes into consideration your race, sex and age. Even though your serum creatinine is in the normal range, you may have kidney disease. Being proactive and discussing your risk for kidney disease with your doctor may help you prevent further injury to your kidneys.

Creatinine is a protein produced by muscle and released into the blood. Normal levels are 0.6 to 1.0 mg/dL (milligrams per deci-liter). The amount of creatinine produced per day is relatively constant. The creatinine level in the serum is determined by the rate it is removed by the kidney. As kidney function decreases, serum creatinine levels increase.

Although kidney function is now determined by a computer program in most laboratories, a simple formula (what we used before we had fancy computer programs) can be used to help us understand the relationship between blood creatinine and kidney function. The old formula, called the Cockcroft-Gault formula, can be used to give an approximate estimation of kidney function (KF) if we know your ideal body weight

(IBW) in kilograms (2.2 pounds equal one kilogram), age, and your serum creatinine level (Cr)

Kidney Function = KF

KF = (140 - age) x IBW divided by (Cr x 72)

For example, if a 75 year old male who weighs 60 kilograms (kg) and has a serum creatinine of 4.0 mg/dL:

KF = (140 – 75) x 60 kg divided by (4 x 72)
    = 13.5 %

This means that this man's kidney function is less than 15% or he has lost more than 85% of his normal kidney function.

Using the same example and different serum creatinine levels we find out that Kidney Function decrease as serum creatinine increases.

75 year old male who weighs 60 kg

Creatinine (mg/dL)	Kidney Function (%)
1.0	54.6
2.0	27.3
3.0	18.0
4.0	13.5

40 year old male who weights 80 kg

Creatinine (mg/dL)	Kidney Function (%)
1.0	111.1
2.0	55.5
3.0	37.0
4.0	27.7
5.0	22.2
6.0	18.5
7.0	15.8

Note that kidney function decreases with increasing age and increases with increasing weight. Younger people have better kidney function than older people. Therefore, as we get older, we all will lose some kidney function. Kidney function is better with increased weight because, for most people, the more we weigh the more muscle we have. The more muscle you have the more creatinine your body will produce. A 40 year old man will not need to start dialysis until his creatinine is over 7.0 mg/dL where a man of 70 years of age will start dialysis when his creatinine is 4.0 mg/dl.

There are many internet sources to help you determine your exact kidney function. One of the best is found on the web site http://www.kdoqi.org. This website has useful information on kidney disease and guidelines for treatment. On this web site you will find a section called GFR calculator. GFR stands for Glomerular Filtration Rate and refers to the kidneys (which is made up of many small glomeruli) ability to filter and clean blood. The computer calculation of GFR can be determined from a serum creatinine level (in milligrams per deciliter), your race (black or white) and your gender (male or female).

Once you have determined your kidney function, you can then determine your stage of kidney disease. Shown below is the nationally recognized staging for kidney diseases.

Stage	Description	Percent Function
One	Minimal injury	Greater than 90%
Two	Mild injury	60 – 89%
Three	Moderate injury	30 – 59%
Four	Severe injury	15 – 29%
Five	Kidney failure	Less than 15%

Once you know your Kidney Function (KF) you can easily determine what stage of kidney disease you have based on your current Creatinine (Cr).

The 40 year old man described above would move into Stage Two disease when his Cr rose above 1.5 mg/dL. As stated above, he would enter Stage Five when his Cr became greater than 7.0 mg/dL.

40 year old male who weights 80 kg

Cr mg/dL	KF (%)	Stage	Description
1.0	111.1	One	Minimal injury
1.5	74.1	Two	Mild injury
2.0	55.5	Three	Moderate injury
4.0	27.7	Four	Severe injury
7.0	15.8	Five	Kidney failure

Simple Formula for Percent Kidney Function (SPKF)

$$SPKF = \frac{(140 - Age)}{Cr}$$

If Age = 40, then SPFK= 140 – 40/Cr = 100/Cr
Cr = 1   SPKF = 100/1 = 100%
Cr = 2   SPKF = 100/2 = 50%
Cr = 3   SPKF = 100/3 = 33%
Cr = 4   SPKF = 100/4 = 25%
Cr = 5   SPKF = 100/5 = 20%

Why is kidney therapy so important?

Kidney protective therapy is a term used to describe therapies that have been shown to slow down kidney disease progression. Let me now explain what that means. The kidney is made up of small filtration units called glomeruli. Each one is like a small kidney. Each one contains very small blood vessels that help to filter blood and excrete waste products. Each one produces hormones. In a single kidney, there are about one million glomeruli. If we took a biopsy of kidneys at various stages of kidney disease we would see that as kidney function decreases, some glomeruli become scarred and no longer function. In simple terms, this means that if a person's kidney function is at 40%, 60% of the kidney function has been lost or 60% of the glomeruli have been scarred. Shown below, is a cartoon demonstrating this concept. Each rectangle contains five glomeruli. As kidney disease progresses from mild disease to kidney failure, more gomeruli are scarred (circles filled in with black). Glomeruli that are healthy are represented by circles not filled in with black.

Stages of Kidney Disease

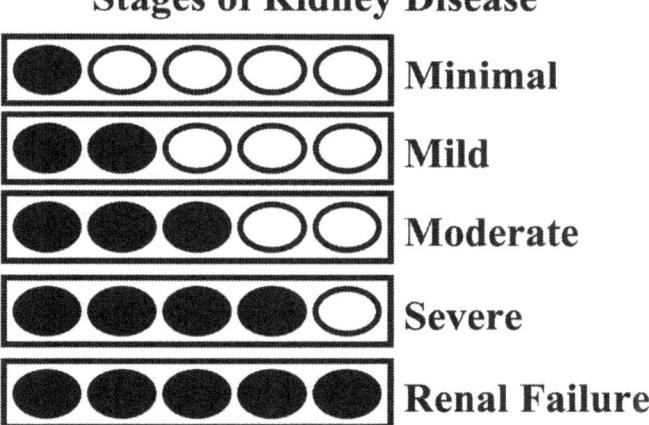

Our goal with kidney protective therapy is to slow down kidney disease progression. The beneficial effect is a delay for the need of dialysis to treat kidney failure.

As shown in the cartoon below, with kidney function as a percent of normal kidney function on the vertical axis and years of age on the horizontal axis, late intervention therapy or late kidney protective treatment for kidney disease results in dialysis therapy being required to maintain life at age 55. If this same person receives early intervention therapy or early kidney protective therapy we can delay the need for dialysis until the person is 80 years or older.

Kidney Disease Prevention

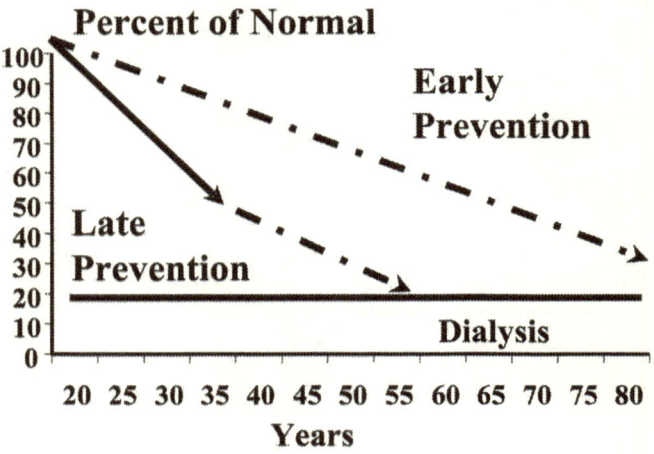

Because the medical community has seen the potential of kidney disease preventive therapy, there is a need now more than ever to get this information out to the general population. Slowing down progression of kidney disease means less cost for the individual with kidney disease (co-pays, hospitalizations, and medications), less cost for society, and lowering of health care premiums. By being proactive and saving your kidneys, you may also be saving yourself thousands of dollars and saving your life.

The next cartoon demonstrates this point. In March of 2004, a group of doctors looking at data from a large Health Maintenance Organization (HMO) reported five year follow up data on over 27,000 patients with Chronic Kidney Disease (CKD). The conclusions were very interesting. The good news was people with Stage Two (CKD 2) or Stage Three (CKD 3) only had about a one percent chance of needing dialysis over a five year period. The bad news was their mortality rate was about twenty percent over a five year period. The news was worse for people with Stage Four (CKD 4) kidney diseases. These people had about a twenty percent chance of needing dialysis in five years but a mortality rate of almost fifty percent over the same period of time. This means that almost one-half of the people in Stage Four would die over a five year period before they ever needed dialysis.

This data strongly suggests that we should take kidney disease very seriously and aggressive therapy should be offered to all patients with kidney disease. Our goal is not just to prevent dialysis but to save lives by preventing people from entering Stage Four kidney disease.

Five Year CKD Follow Up Study
Archives of Internal Medicine
Volume 164 (6), March 22, 2004, Pages 659663

	RRT	Death
CKD 2	1.1%	19.5%
CKD 3	1.3%	24.3%
CKD 4	19.9%	45.7%

RRT = Renal Replacement Therapy
N = 27,998 HMO patients

Reduce the pressure inside the kidneys

All patients with kidney disease should be on medications that will lower the pressure inside the vessels of the kidney and the millions of tiny filtration units of the kidney called glomeruli. These medications lower pressure in the kidney by blocking the effects of the renin-angiotensin system.

The renin-angiotensin system is a hormone feedback system in your body that plays an important role in regulating blood volume, arterial pressure, and pressure inside the kidneys. While the pathways for this system have been found in a number of tissues, the most important site for release of these regulating hormones is the kidney. Nervous system stimulation, renal artery hypotension, and decreased sodium delivery to the kidney stimulate the release of renin by the kidney.

Renin is an enzyme that cuts a large protein called angiotensinogen, which is made in the liver, into a smaller protein called Angiotensin I (AI). Cells on the walls of blood vessels, particularly in the lungs, contain another enzyme called Angiotensin Converting Enzyme (ACE) that converts angiotensin I to angiotensin II (AII). Angiotensin II has several important functions which include:

- Constricts blood vessels inside and outside the kidney.
- Stimulates the release of aldosterone from the adrenal gland which causes the kidneys to increase sodium or salt absorption.
- Stimulates the brain to release vasopressin which causes the kidneys to increase fluid retention.

Angiotensin II is a very powerful protein molecule that raises blood pressure throughout the body by the mechanisms stated above. After years of research, two types of medications called Angiotensin Converting Enzyme Inhibitors (ACEI) and Angiotensin Receptor Blockers (ARB) were developed to block the effects of AII.

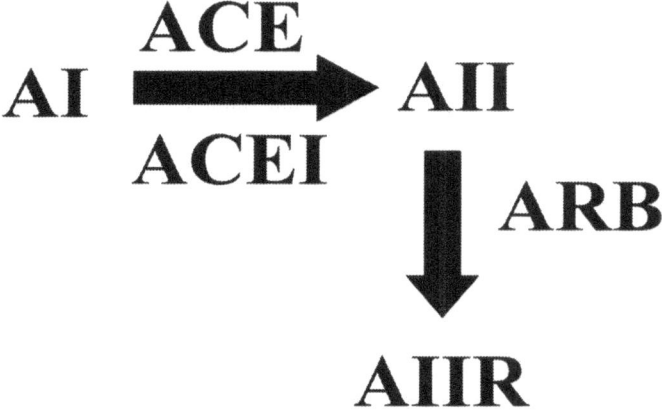

As shown in the cartoon above, ACEI blocks ACE and therefore prevents the formation of AII. As a result, the body makes more AI and can theoretically override the ACEI system leading to some formation of AII. ARB blocks the receptor site on blood vessels that serves as the docking space for AII. No matter how much AI is produced it cannot bind to the receptor. ARBs are theoretically a better medication because they block the effects of AII, downstream. As a result, blood pressure is lowered and the body is protected from the effect of a high pressure system. Studies using these medications demonstrated a side effect that was unexpected. In addition to lowering the systemic blood pressure, ACEI and ARBs slowed down the progression of kidney disease in patients with diabetes.

This led to the term reno-protective or kidney protective therapy. These medications are now the medications of choice for patients with kidney disease or who have the potential for developing kidney disease.

As shown below, the normal anatomy of the glomerulus includes small arteries that bring blood to the glomerulus (A) and small arteries that take blood away from the glomerulus (B). This would be similar to a water balloon that has an entrance port (A) and an exit port (B). When AII levels rise they bind to receptors on the small arteries leaving the glomerulus (B), causing the small artery to get smaller and increasing "back" pressure to the kidney. As shown in the cartoon, this effect is like blowing air into a balloon at port A and then pinching port B with your fingers. As a result, pressure increases inside the balloon and the balloon gets bigger.

Anatomy of Glomerulus

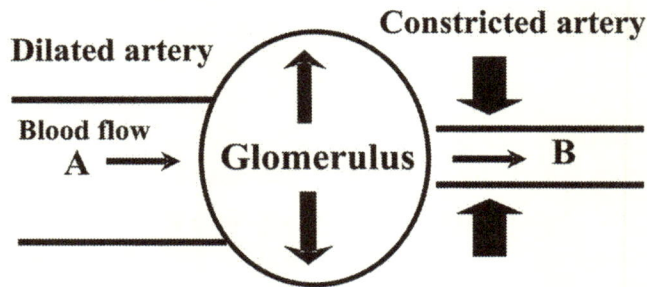

**AII causes constriction of
arteries leaving glomerulus (B)
causing an increase in pressure inside the glomerulus**

In the next cartoon, I show the changes that occur after initiation of ACEI or ARB therapy. ACEI and ARB block the effects of AII on the small arteries leaving the kidney (B). As a result, the small arteries dilate or get larger and pressure decreases inside the glomerulus. Using the balloon example, this would be like blowing air into the balloon at port A and releasing pressure at port B. The pressure inside the balloon would decrease and the balloon would get smaller.

Anatomy of Glomerulus

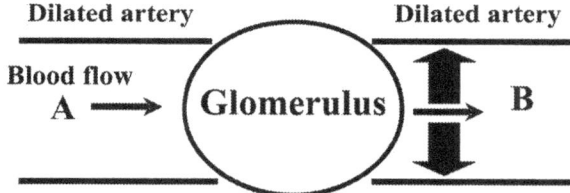

**AECEI and ARB block constriction
of arteries leaving the glomerulus (B)
causing a decrease in pressure inside the glomerulus**

Reduce the pressure outside the kidney

High blood pressure occurs when the pressure of your blood against the walls of your blood vessels increases. If uncontrolled, high blood pressure can lead to heart attack, stroke, and kidney disease. Data from hypertension registries suggest that we are not doing a good job of controlling hypertension. Only about 50% of Americans with hypertension have their blood pressure controlled with treatment. More alarming, was a recent study released in the journal "Stroke," which showed that Americans with "pre-hypertension" (120/80 to 139/89 mmHg) were three times more likely to have a heart attack than Americans with normal blood pressure.

Hypertension is a common health issue in the United States. High blood pressure increases the pressure outside the kidney which eventually leads to kidney damage. It is estimated that 20 percent of the general population has hypertension and 65 percent of patients over 65 have hypertension. Hypertension is defined as a blood pressure greater than 140/90 mmHg. Optimal blood pressure for people with kidney disease is a blood pressure less than 130/80 mmHg. Lifestyle changes that decrease blood pressure include weight loss, low salt diet, exercise and limited alcohol intake. Despite knowing these facts, blood pressure is not well controlled and millions of patients are presently taking blood pressure medications. Most patients with hypertension (95 percent) have hypertension of unknown etiology. Other individuals have what is called secondary hypertension.

Common causes of secondary hypertension include birth control pills, anti-histamine medication, kidney disease, thyroid disease, and tumors secreting hormones that raise the blood pressure. The treatment of hypertension can be difficult in a patient who is resistant to standardize therapy. First line treatment for hypertension is always a low sodium diet, weight loss, and exercise. Low sodium diet appears to be particularly helpful in elderly and African American individuals. Weight loss and exercise is helpful in almost all patients. All patients with high blood pressure should stop tobacco use and limit alcohol intake to no more than two drinks per day.

A low sodium diet is very important in controlling blood pressure. Sodium intake causes the body to retain water. Increased sodium and water in our blood vessels elevates our blood pressure. By limiting our sodium intake or increasing the kidney removal of salt (via water pills) we can lower our blood pressure. Sodium is present in almost all foods prepared at fast food restaurants. Hidden sources of salt are found in seasonings (garlic salt), pickled foods, canned vegetables and soups, packaged foods, and luncheon meats. Packaged foods contain information of their sodium content. We ask individuals with high blood pressure to try and limit their daily sodium intake to less than 2,000 milligrams or 2 grams per day. For reference, some soup products contain 800 to 1000 mg of sodium per cup. Most individuals are surprised how much salt they ingest every day.

Sodium is a mineral or electrolyte that is involved in both electrical and cellular functions in the body. Normal kidneys remove excess sodium from the body and excrete the excess sodium into the urine. When kidney function decreases, sodium consumed in our diet is not removed by the kidneys and may remain in the body.

Excess sodium in the body is associated with water retention and secondary swelling of extremities often called edema. Excess sodium in the body can cause increased thirst, tissue swelling, high blood pressure, and heart failure. Most people with kidney failure should be on a low sodium diet. A low sodium diet means you can consume about 2 grams (2000 mg) of sodium per day. Avoid extra sodium in your diet if you are short of breath or observe swelling of your legs or hands. Remember that water goes where sodium goes. Always seek medical attention if you are short of breath.

Sodium content of common foods	
Food	**Sodium**
One teaspoon table salt	2000 mg (2 grams)
One slice of lunch meat	300 mg
One hot dog	500 mg
One cup of soup	900 mg
One pickle (large)	1430 mg
One large slice of pizza	600 mg
One diet soda (12 ounces)	75 mg
One bread slice	150 mg
One teaspoon butter	30 mg
One tablespoon salad dressing	160 mg

In America, the average individual may ingest over 8,000 mg of sodium daily. When you start a low sodium diet do not get discouraged. Most people, will notice that food just does not taste the same. This is because we have been eating high sodium diets for most of our lives. Over time, your body (and taste buds) will adjust. The benefit is that you may not have to take blood pressure medications or if you are on blood pressure medications you may not have to take as much medication as someone who does not follow a low sodium diet. Less medication means fewer side effects.

Second line therapy in people without kidney disease is usually a diuretic (water pill). Diuretics help treat hypertension by helping our bodies excrete salt. Side effects of diuretics include lower serum potassium levels (form potassium wasting) and an elevation of your serum glucose levels. Low serum potassium levels may irritate your heart or give you feelings of fatigue or weakness. Elevated serum blood sugar could predispose you to diabetes mellitus. Additional medications used to treat hypertension include beta blockers and calcium channel blockers. These medications prevent blood vessel constriction and allow blood vessels to relax resulting in a lower blood pressure. The main side effects of beta-blockers include feeling tired and slow heart rate. Calcium channel blockers side effects include constipation, leg swelling, headache, and a low heart rate.

Most people's blood pressure can be controlled with two blood pressure medications. Some individuals need three medications, which most often include a water pill and additional medications. Blood pressure can be controlled by teamwork. You should invest in a home blood pressure monitoring system that allows you to check your blood pressure daily. Record your blood pressure measurements and share this information with your healthcare professional team at each medical visit. Monitor your blood pressure on a regular basis. Contact you health care professional if your blood pressure is consistently greater than 140/90 mmHg. By obtaining control of your blood pressure, you will significantly reduce your risk of developing kidney disease, heart disease and stroke.

People with severe kidney disease may require the use of as many as four different types of blood pressure medication to control blood pressure. The regimen used may include kidney protective medication like ACEI and ARB, an alpha beta blocker, a calcium channel blocker and a vasodilator. If blood pressure is still not controlled a work up should be initiated to rule out secondary hypertension.

The workup for secondary hypertension requires a series of blood tests and radiological scans. The most common cause of secondary hypertension is over-the-counter medication (non-steroidal anti-inflammatory medications, birth control pills and anti-histamines), chronic kidney disease, renal artery stenosis, thyroid disease and adrenal gland tumors that secrete hormones which raise the blood pressure. Most of these conditions can be ruled out by obtaining serum thyroid hormone levels, urine cortisol levels, urine aldosterone hormone levels and a CT scan of abdomen. If all these tests are negative then your physician may ask you to do a test to rule out renal artery stenosis.

Renal artery stenosis is a narrowing or blockage of the artery that supplies blood to the kidney. The disease is caused by fibromuscular dysplasia (common in young females) or atherosclerosis (common in older men). In fibromuscular dysplasia, the artery is occluded by a congenital disease which causes the renal artery wall to thicken. In atherosclerosis, plaques or cholesterol deposits occlude the artery. Renal artery stenosis causes hypertension by decreasing blood flow to the kidneys. The kidney thinks that the blood pressure is low so it makes a hormone called renin that causes the blood pressure to increase. The diagnosis of renal artery stenosis is made by an arteriogram. In this study, dye is injected into the renal artery and pictures are taken of the vessel. Blood samples are also taken from the blood vessels and measured for renin. If the vessel is closing, a specialist can open the artery with a small balloon. When the renal artery is opened, blood flow is returned to the kidney and the kidney no longer thinks the blood pressure is low. The kidney stops making renin and blood pressure returns to normal.

Prevent damage inside the kidney

The best way to prevent damage inside the kidney is to control diabetes (if you have diabetes), treat high cholesterol levels (if your cholesterol levels are elevated) and know your medications.

Treat diabetes aggressively.

Since 1990, there has been a 33% increase in number of diabetics. The sharpest rise was among people in their thirties. Diabetes is the number one cause of blindness, amputation, and kidney failure.

Most people on dialysis are there because of diabetes. Diabetes consumes 25% of annual Medicare costs. For the most part, Type 2 diabetes is preventable through diet and exercise. A recent study showed that preventive care decreases the complications of diabetes by as much as 50% (imagine 50% less diabetics on dialysis). It is estimated that unless we change our present life-style, one-third of our children will develop diabetes in their lifetime.

Individuals with diabetes mellitus are at risk for developing kidney disease. In diabetes mellitus, the body does not make enough insulin to keep blood sugar levels normal. Uncontrolled diabetes mellitus with constantly elevated blood sugars can result in blindness (diabetic retinopathy), loss of feeling in the legs (diabetic neuropathy) and kidney disease (diabetic nephropathy). For this reason, individuals with diabetes mellitus need to monitor and control blood sugars.

The metabolic syndrome characterized by obesity and elevated blood sugars can also lead to kidney disease. In these individuals, weight loss and following a diabetic diet are crucial to their long-term survival and prevention from getting kidney disease.

To control blood sugars, it is important to follow a diabetic diet, exercise regularly and monitor blood sugars daily. A dietician can help you design a diet that is right for you. Blood sugar monitoring is usually done with a glucose-monitoring machine. These are available through your health care provider. Blood sugars should normally be less than 120 mg/dl.

Blood sugar levels greater than 150 mg/dl is abnormal. Your health care provider may monitor you blood sugar control by performing a lab test called the HgbA1C level. This test lets you know how well your blood sugar has been controlled the last few months. Normal HgbA1C levels are less than 6%. An individual with uncontrolled diabetes mellitus could have HgbA1C levels greater than 10%. For individuals who cannot control their blood sugars with diet, exercise and weight loss, medications or insulin may be needed. Your health care professional will determine the medication regimen that is right for you. If you have kidney disease, diabetes medications may need to be adjusted based on your kidney function tests. In general, insulin therapy is safe for individuals with kidney disease. Since the kidneys metabolize insulin, less insulin therapy may be needed to control blood sugar levels as kidney function deteriorates. Also as kidney function deteriorates, your health care professional may want to change you from long acting medications used to treat diabetes that may accumulate in your body to short acting medications that are metabolized quickly. Long acting blood sugar lowering medications may severely lower blood sugar levels and cause you to go into a hypoglycemic or low blood sugar coma. As your kidney function deteriorates, discuss adjusting your diabetes treatment regimen with your health care professional.

Treat high cholesterol levels

LDL cholesterol is called the "bad cholesterol" because it takes cholesterol from the liver and deposits cholesterol on blood vessels throughout your body. High levels of LDL cholesterol are associated with a high mortality rate secondary to coronary artery disease. Most Americans now understand the importance on controlling blood cholesterol levels. Most Americans know their cholesterol level and if it is elevated have been advised to lower their intake of high cholesterol foods and possibly take cholesterol-lowering medications. A low cholesterol diet involves limiting intake of foods that are high in cholesterol. This includes decreasing intake of red meats and eggs. Over the counter egg products that do not contain the yolk of the egg are good sources of protein and do not raise your blood cholesterol level. For individuals who are not able to control their blood cholesterol level with diet, they may want to seek consultation with their health care provider and ask about starting therapy with cholesterol lowering agents.

There are many types of cholesterol lowering medications and your health care provider will determine which one is right for you. Your target cholesterol goal to decrease risk of kidney disease progression is to lower your low-density lipoprotein or LDL cholesterol to less than 100 mg/dl.

Know your medications

Many medications are toxic to the kidneys. Individuals with kidney disease or who are at risk for developing kidney disease should be aware of all medications that may injure the kidney. The most common cause of kidney injury by an over the counter medication is a group of medications called non-steroidal anti-inflammatory medications. These are commonly known as ibuprofen and naproxen. If you have kidney disease, these medications should be avoided at all costs. If you have pain and need pain medications consider taking acetaminophen until you can discuss pain management with your health care professional.

Other medications that may injure the kidneys include contrast dye used for radiological studies, antibiotics, and herbs. Contrast dye is a direct kidney toxin. This dye is used during radiological procedures to look at blood flow to the heart, brain, liver, and kidneys. Large amounts of contrast dye can cause acute renal failure. Individuals with kidney disease, heart failure and diabetes mellitus are at risk for this type of renal injury. If you have any of these conditions please inform the radiology department staff that you may be at risk for contrast induced kidney injury. Other options include a MRI, which uses a contrast material that is not toxic to the kidneys.

Antibiotics can cause allergic reactions that may affect the kidneys. Similarly, some can cause scarring and irreversible kidney damage. If you have kidney disease, inform your health care professional about the need to adjust antibiotic dosing based on your kidney function. In general all patients with kidney disease are advised to avoid herbal treatment until they have discussed possible side effects with their health care professional.

In addition to increasing awareness about medications that can hurt your kidneys there are medications that can protect your kidneys. These medications are called kidney or renal protective medications and they help preserve kidney function by decreasing the pressure on the kidneys. Most renal protective medications are also used to treat high blood pressure. These medications work by preventing the formation and binding of substances that cause blood vessels in the kidney to constrict. As a result, blood pressure is lowered inside the kidney and the kidney is protected. These medications have been shown to slow down progression of renal disease and extend the life of the kidney and delay the time when individuals with kidney disease need to start dialysis therapy. All patients with kidney disease and all patients with diabetes mellitus should be evaluated by their health care provider as candidates for this type of protective therapy.

Finally, all patients with kidney disease (and all individuals) should avoid tobacco products. Tobacco serves no useful purpose in life. Smoking cigarettes causes irreversible changes in your lung cells and the cells lining the blood vessels of the brain, heart and kidneys. If you smoke you lose. Just stop smoking.

Medications that may require dose modification in kidney failure

Medication	Examples
Heart drugs	digoxin
Antibiotics	penicillin,ciprofloxacin,sulfa, nitrofurantoin
Anti-viral	acyclovir
Anti-fungal	fluconazole
Anti-gout	allopurinol

Medications to avoid in kidney failure

Medication	Examples
Anti-ulcer	cimetidine
Stool softeners	all products containing phosphate, magnesium, or aluminum
Diuretics (water pills)	potassium sparing diuretics
Pain Medications	NSAIDS
Radiology	dyes used for radiology and heart studies

IV. Complications of Kidney Disease

Prevent malnutrition

Serum albumin is a protein in our blood that is made in the liver and important for normal body functions. Low serum albumin or low body protein stores is called malnutrition and can result in poor healing and decreased immunity, which can make us susceptible to infections. Low blood protein or low serum albumin levels are associated with a high mortality rate.

The mortality rate of End Stage Renal Disease (ESRD) in the United States is approximately 20% per year (US RDS). Since efforts to treat cardiovascular diseases and dialysis inadequacy have not significantly reduced mortality of ESRD, researchers are looking for other causes for poor dialysis outcomes. Protein malnutrition, which occurs frequently in ESRD, may be one of the most important causes of the high rate of mortality in ESRD. Studies have shown a strong correlation between mortality and malnutrition in ESRD with mortality rates increasing as serum albumin levels decrease. Protein malnutrition appears to precede dialysis treatment as shown in the Modification of Diet in Renal Disease Study. Inadequate protein intake and inflammation may be the two most important causes of malnutrition in kidney disease.

The most common cause of protein malnutrition is probably a decreased appetite from progression of kidney disease and build-up of kidney toxins. Other causes of malnutrition in kidney disease may include diabetes gastroparesis, depression, dietary restrictions (low protein diet), and inability to get good nutrition (low income, physical disability, mental disability). In some cases, protein malnutrition is associated with socioeconomic status.

Another important cause of malnutrition is chronic inflammation as characterized by an elevation in C-reactive protein. Possible causes of inflammation include coronary artery disease, malignancy, systemic inflammatory diseases, and infections (dental infections, tuberculosis and urinary tract infections).

Inflammation causes a problem in the mobilization of the proteins absorbed in our diet into adequate protein stores in our blood. The low blood protein results in poor blood vessel healing, which in turn causes low blood protein levels. The process perpetuates itself into a cascade of events, which results in chronically low blood protein levels that is not improved by increasing protein intake in the diet. At this time, it is unclear if malnutrition causes inflammation (poor wound healing and impaired immune response) or inflammation causes malnutrition (decrease in appetite, increased protein breakdown, and vascular injury).

Patients with very high levels of inflammation are at most risk for death. These patients should be monitored closely and an aggressive search for inflammation should be initiated (coronary artery disease testing, foot exam in diabetes mellitus, dental exam, blood and urine cultures, serology for hepatitis). Although studies strongly link inflammation to poor outcome in kidney disease, there are no randomized clinical trials to indicate improvement in ESRD mortality by inflammation-reducing approaches.

Possible treatment modalities to help manage inflammation include identifying and treating the underlying cause and initiation of treatment modalities that may reduce inflammation. Examples include use of angiotensin-converting enzyme inhibitors, cholesterol lowering agents (statins) and vitamin E. Patients with low serum albumin levels and normal levels of C reactive protein may have inadequate protein intake. Initial investigations should include a protein intake assessment and a determination of twenty-four hour urine urea nitrogen. The urine urea nitrogen is a useful indicator of the dietary protein intake. Low levels indicate inadequate protein intake while high levels indicate adequate protein intake.

Solving the malnutrition problem in kidney disease involves developing a treatment plan to improve and control nutritional outcomes. The results of interventions used to improve blood protein levels can take weeks or months to see improvement. The first step is to try and understand the cause of low blood protein. Most patients do not know they are malnourished, so education is an important part of the treatment. Many patients probably do not get enough protein in their diet. Some cannot afford foods that contain high quality protein and others do not have time to prepare nutritious meals.

Malnourished patients can increase blood protein levels by consuming foods that contain large amounts of high biological protein such as tofu, meat and eggs. These foods contain the essential amino acids which are crucial for humans to synthesize proteins in their bodies. However, meat and eggs may not be good for people with chronic kidney disease because they contain high levels of cholesterol. Protein supplements including those which contain all the essential amino acids may be a good alternative.

Some protein supplements (protein powders, protein drinks or protein bars) are safe for individuals with kidney disease and others are not. Individuals with kidney disease should avoid protein supplements that contain large amounts of phosphorus, potassium, or cholesterol. Not all protein supplements are the same so you need to talk to a dietician before taking over the counter supplements that may be harmful to your body. Our goal should be to assure that no patient with kidney disease suffers from malnutrition.

Daily protein requirement by weight		
Weight		**Protein requirement**
Kg	**Pounds**	**Grams per day**
50	110	75
60	132	90
70	154	105
80	176	120
90	198	135
100	220	150
110	242	165
120	264	180
130	286	195

Protein Source	**Protein per unit dose (estimate)**
Meat	7 grams of protein per ounce
Eggs	7 grams of protein per egg
No yolk eggs	25 grams of protein per cup
Protein powder	5 grams of protein per scoop
Protein drink	15 grams of protein per can
Protein bars	15 grams of protein per bar

Prevent anemia

Anemia is defined as having less than a normal number of red blood cells or less than normal hemoglobin in the blood. Hemoglobin is a red pigment that gives the red color to red blood cells and to blood. Hemoglobin is the key chemical compound that combines with oxygen from the lungs and carries the oxygen from the lungs to cells throughout the body. Oxygen is essential for cells to produce energy. When hemoglobin is low, oxygen transport through the body is low. The person with anemia is under-oxygenated and may complain about feeling tired, and becoming short of breath with exercise. Anemia is caused by low levels of iron in the blood and/or a decrease in production of a hormone called EPO.

People who are iron deficient usually have blood tests that show their total body iron stores have been depleted. Two tests commonly used to determine body iron stores are transferrin saturation and blood ferritin levels. A person is considered iron deficient if their transferrin saturation level is less than 20% and a blood ferritin level is less than 100 ng/ml.

The normal kidney produces a hormone called erythropoietin or EPO. This hormone is secreted when hemoglobin in the blood starts to decrease. When individuals get kidney disease, erythropoietin production is diminished. Patients with anemia related to chronic kidney disease can be treated with erythropoietin shots.

Prevent bone disease

Calcium is one the most common minerals in the human body. Ninety-nine percent of the calcium in your body is found in your bones. About one percent is found in the blood and soft tissues of your body. Calcium levels in the blood and fluid surrounding the cells must be maintained within a very narrow range for normal functioning of the heart, brain, muscles and bones.

The normal kidney makes Vitamin D. In kidney disease, Vitamin D is not produced and deficiency of Vitamin D results in decreased absorption of calcium and phosphorus from the gastrointestinal tract. As serum calcium levels fall, the body secretes a hormone called Parathyroid Hormone (PTH) from the parathyroid gland located on either side of your thyroid glands in your neck.

Parathyroid hormone is the most important endocrine regulator of calcium and phosphorus concentration in the body. This hormone finds its major target cells in the bones and kidneys. The hormones main job is to increase serum calcium levels and decrease serum phosphorus levels. Vitamin D in the blood suppresses secretion of parathyroid hormone.

Parathyroid hormone causes bone to release calcium and phosphorus into the blood. The hormone also increases production of Vitamin D and increases the kidney's ability to get rid of phosphorus into the urine. Vitamin D is not produced in people with chronic kidney disease so calcium and phosphorus are poorly absorbed in the gut. The kidney cannot excrete phosphorus so serum phosphorus levels rise.

Parathyroid hormone levels rise to maintain normal calcium levels and decrease elevated phosphorus levels. As parathyroid hormone levels rise, bone breakdown occurs at an accelerated rate. Uncontrolled bone breakdown can result in weak bones and fractures. The parathyroid gland does not know when the kidneys are not working well. Since the kidney does not make Vitamin D, parathyroid hormone secretion is not inhibited.

Phosphorus is an essential mineral that is required by every cell in the body for normal functioning. The majority of the phosphorus in the body is found as phosphate. Approximately 85% of the body's phosphorus is found in bone. Normal body phosphorus levels are required for energy production. Elevated calcium and phosphorus levels can cause calcification of tissues leading to organ damage and heart disease.

In kidney disease, it is important to keep parathyroid hormone levels and serum phosphorus levels in normal range. We can decrease parathyroid hormone levels by taking oral or intravenous Vitamin D. Foods that are high in phosphorus and should be limited if your phosphate levels are high include dairy products (milk, cheese, yogurt), nuts and seeds, beans and peas, bran cereals and bran muffins, and colas and beer. Eating a low phosphorus diet and taking phosphate binders with your meals normalizes phosphorus levels. If your blood levels of phosphorus become elevated, you can take medications that bind phosphorus in the gut and lower blood phosphorus levels. Examples of commonly used phosphate binders include calcium carbonate, calcium acetate, and sevelamar. Unless otherwise instructed by your physician, try to maintain a serum phosphorus level less than 5.5 mg/dl and a parathyroid hormone level less than 180 pg/ml.

Foods that are high in phosphorus (foods to avoid)
Dairy products: milk, cheese, yogurt, cream soup
Fruits and vegetables: asparagus, peas, mushrooms, corn, beans, dried beans, prunes
Breads: bran muffins, pancakes, waffles, whole wheat bread, pizza, corn bread, bran cereals
Nuts, peanut butter, and seeds
Chocolate and cocoa
Dark colored beverages (colas and beer)

Prevent hyperkalemia

Potassium is a mineral or electrolyte that is involved in both electrical and cellular functions in the body. Potassium plays a role in keeping your heartbeat regular and your muscles working properly. It is the job of the kidneys to keep the right amount of potassium in your body. When kidneys no longer work well it is difficult for the body to get rid of potassium. Patients with kidney disease are unable to excrete excess potassium into their urine. High levels of potassium in our blood or hyperkalemia can result in cardiac arrhythmias and sudden death.

The recommended daily allowance for potassium is 2-3 grams per day for individuals with kidney disease. Elevated blood potassium can be caused by decreased excretion of potassium from the body (kidney disease and some medications) or increased intake of high potassium foods (see below). If your blood potassium levels are high avoid foods that are very high in potassium. Potassium can be removed from your body by taking medications that bind potassium in the gut. Hemodialysis may be needed to treat very high blood potassium levels in emergency situations.

Foods high in potassium (foods to avoid)
Salt substitutes: potassium chloride
Dairy products: milk, yogurt, cheeses
Whole grains: breads, cereals, muffins
Starchy vegetables: potatoes, dried beans, yams, winter squash
Other vegetables: tomatoes, broccoli, peas, lima beans, spinach
Fruits: bananas, oranges, citrus fruits, apricots

Prevent Hepatitis B infections

Hepatitis means inflammation of the liver and is usually secondary to a virus called Hepatitis B. Hepatitis B virus infections are usually caused by exposure to blood of someone with Hepatitis B viral infection. Because kidney disease patients are at risk to receive a blood transfusion sometime in their lives, all patients with kidney disease are advised to get immunized with a vaccine that will decrease their chance of developing Hepatitis B infection.

The success of immunizing you with Hepatitis B vaccine depends on where you are in the kidney disease spectrum. Before someone goes into renal failure the chance of successful immunization, as determined by the formation of hepatitis B antibodies in your blood, is about 90%. Once someone develops kidney failure the success rate drops to 50%. Finally, if they get a kidney transplant the success rate is a dismal 10%. This is why we want to immunize you now.

The Hepatitis B vaccination is a little different than the flu vaccine. The flu vaccine is designed to expose you to many different types of viruses. The Hepatitis B vaccine exposes you to one type of a dead virus. The immunization does not usually produce a flu-like response. Most people do not complain of having a reaction after the Hepatitis B vaccine.

V. Kidney Replacement Therapy

Individuals with kidney failure are informed that when your kidneys fail you will need renal replacement therapy to sustain life. When someone is diagnosed as having renal failure their options include starting dialysis, transplantation, or no treatment.

Hemodialysis

In the United States, 90% of renal failure patients who have not had a kidney transplant are on hemodialysis. Hemodialysis cleans and filters your blood using a machine to temporarily rid your body of harmful wastes, extra salt, and extra water. Hemodialysis uses a special filter called a dialyzer that functions as an artificial kidney to clean your blood. During treatment, your blood travels through tubes into the dialyzer, which filters out wastes and extra water. Cleaned blood flows through another set of tubes back into your body. The dialyzer is connected to a machine that monitors blood flow and removes wastes from the blood. Dialysis is usually needed three times a week to keep your blood free of toxins and excess fluid. Each treatment lasts from 3 to 5 hours. During dialysis treatment, you can read, write, sleep, talk, or watch television.

Before starting hemodialysis, you will need a physician to create an access to your blood stream. You may need to stay overnight in the hospital, but many patients have their access placed on an outpatient basis. This access provides an efficient way for blood to be carried from your body to the dialysis machine and back without causing discomfort. The three main types of access are a fistula, graft, or catheter.

To create a fistula, a surgeon connects an artery in your arm to a vein in your arm. The increased blood flow makes the vein grow larger and stronger so that it can be used for repeated needle insertions. This is the preferred type of access because this form of vascular access uses your own blood vessels and does not involve foreign body material. As a result there are fewer infections or problems with clotting. This access may take several weeks or months to heal before it is ready for use

A graft connects an artery to a vein by using a synthetic tube. Grafts develop faster than a fistula so it can be used soon after placement. Because they contain synthetic material, grafts are more likely to have problems with infection and clotting.

If your kidney disease has progressed quickly, you may not have time to get a permanent vascular access before you start dialysis treatments. You may need to use a catheter, a tube inserted into a vein in your neck, chest, or leg near the groin, as a temporary access. Some people use a catheter for long-term access as well. Catheters that will be needed for more than about 3 weeks are placed under the skin to increase comfort and reduce complications.

Hemodialysis is usually done in a dialysis center by trained professionals. In some parts of the country, it can be done at home with the help of a partner. If you decide to do home dialysis, you and your partner will receive special training. Common problems with dialysis include infection, muscle cramps, low blood pressure, weakness, dizziness, or feeling sick to your stomach. You can avoid many side effects if you follow a proper diet, limit your liquid intake, and take your medications as directed. The diet for renal failure patients involves eating enough protein to avoid malnutrition and watching your potassium, fluid, salt, and phosphorus intake.

Benefits of dialysis include going to a dialysis center for renal replacement therapy. At the dialysis center you will be cared for by trained professionals and have an opportunity to socialize with other patients. Disadvantages of dialysis treatments include visits to the dialysis center three times per week, diet restrictions, and problems with vascular access (infections, clotting, multiple surgeries).

Peritoneal Dialysis

Peritoneal dialysis is another procedure that removes extra water, wastes, and chemicals from your body. This procedure uses the lining of your abdomen (called the peritoneal membrane) to filter your blood. The peritoneal membrane acts as a natural artificial kidney. Prior to starting peritoneal dialysis, a soft tube is inserted by a surgeon into your abdomen. After a few weeks of healing, a dialysis solution (which is a mixture of minerals and sugar dissolved in water) travels through the soft tube into your abdomen. Waste products, chemicals, and extra water from the tiny blood vessels in your peritoneal membrane are drawn into the dialysis solution. After several hours, the used solution is drained from your abdomen through the tube, taking the waste products out of your body. Fresh fluid is then inserted and the whole process is repeated throughout the day. Potential complications of peritoneal dialysis include bowel obstruction, constipation, and infection.

The diet for individuals on peritoneal dialysis is similar to patients on hemodialysis. However, patients on peritoneal dialysis can eat more protein since protein is lost in the peritoneal fluid when it is removed from the body. Patients on peritoneal dialysis have more control over their fluids and have to monitor their calories closely to avoid high blood sugar levels. The solution used for peritoneal dialysis contains high concentrations of sugar that can be absorbed through the peritoneal membrane.

The main benefit of peritoneal dialysis is dialysis therapy at home. The diet is less strict and no needle sticks are required. Traveling is easier. The problems associated with peritoneal dialysis include high risk of infection, weight gain and the need for treatment seven days per week.

Transplantation

The third option for management of renal failure is transplantation. In this procedure, a surgeon places the new kidney inside your lower abdomen and connects the artery and vein of the new kidney to your artery and vein. The new kidney produces urine and cleans your blood similar to your native kidney.

Transplantation may not be for everyone. Some individuals have a condition that would make transplantation dangerous or unlikely to succeed. You may receive a kidney from a member of your family (living related donor), a person who has recently died (deceased donor), or a very close friend (living unrelated donor).

Transplantation is a relatively recent phenomenon. Many of the big developments in the area of kidney transplantation have taken place within the past 50 years. Researchers realized that without treatment, patients with kidney disease would die. The first human to human kidney transplant was performed in 1933. Because doctors did not understand the immune system at that time, the transplanted kidney only worked for about one hour.

In the early 1950's, cortisone like medications were used to suppress the human immune system resulting in some successful kidney transplants. In 1954, Joseph E. Murray and a team from Peter Bent Brigham Hospital in Boston performed the first truly successful kidney transplant from one twin to another. This was done without any immunosuppressive medication. Following this surgical success, more kidney transplants between identical twins were performed. To allow patients with end stage renal disease to receive a kidney from non related donor new approaches were needed to prevent the body from rejecting the donor kidney.

In the 1960's, better techniques for matching a donor kidney and to a recipient's immune system were developed and powerful immunosuppressive agents became available. Combining these techniques, helped decrease the likelihood of renal transplant rejection.

After the discovery of the immunosuppressive agent cyclosporine in 1978, transplantation became widespread and successful. Cyclosporine inhibits white blood cells that are the specific mediators of organ rejection. Because these white blood cells (called lymphocytes) are not activated, the immune system is inhibited and kidneys are not rejected. Since the introduction of cyclosporine, the annual mortality rate for kidney transplant patients is less than 5 percent.

Renal transplant can be risky. Because immune systems are suppressed by transplant medications, patients are at high risk for infections. The side effects of cyclosporine and other medications used to suppress the immune system also include hypertension and malignancy.

Before you can get a kidney transplant, you must fulfill three immunological requirements. First, the donor and you must have compatible blood types. This is the most important matching factor. Second, the proteins on your cells must match up with the protein on the cells of the donor kidney. Third, you must have a negative cross match test in which the cells' from the individual who is donating the kidney is mixed with your blood. If these three tests show no significant incompatibilities, the transplantation can take place.

The benefits of a kidney transplant include fewer diet restrictions and no need for dialysis or needle sticks. Life expectancy is significantly improved.

No treatment

For many people, dialysis and transplantation are not good options and no treatment may be the best life path. If your quality of life is poor and you do not wish to extend your life with artificial kidney treatment you can decide on no treatment. This difficult decision may be made after discussing your options with family members or friends. Even if you decide on no treatment you can always decide to start getting treatment at a later date.

You have the right to refuse or withdraw from dialysis treatment at any time. Some patients will express in writing their wishes by naming a person to speak for them if they cannot talk (Durable Power of Attorney for Health Care) or by stating what treatments they would or would not want (Living Will). In addition to dialysis, patients can choose or refuse other life-sustaining treatments such as cardiopulmonary resuscitation, tube feedings, mechanical or artificial respiration, antibiotics, surgery and blood transfusions.

VI. Conclusion

The purpose of this book is to help you *"Save Your Kidneys,"* and develop a plan to meet your kidney health care goals. In addition, our goal is to help you overcome barriers that prevent you from achieving your kidney health care goals by giving you knowledge about the causes and treatments of kidney disease. By understanding the causes and treatment of kidney disease, you will have the knowledge needed to slow down kidney disease progression and avoid the need for dialysis or transplantation.

If we are successful, we will save kidney function and save lives. Working together we can lower health care costs for you and your family and help you and your family live healthier and longer lives.

VII. References

- Brenner & Rector's The Kidney, 7ᵗʰ ed. Copyright © 2004 Elsevier

- Keith DS, Nichols GA, Gullion, CM, Brown JB, Smith, DH. Longitudinal follow-up and outcomes among a population with chronic kidney disease in a large managed care organization. Archives of Internal Medicine. Volume 164(6) 22 March 2004 p 659–663

- The National Kidney Foundation - Kidney/Disease Outcomes Quality Initiative (NKF-K/DOQI) Clinical practice guidelines for chronic kidney disease: Evaluation, classification, and stratification. Am J Kidney Dis 39:S1-S246, 2002 (suppl 1)

- National Kidney Foundation Kidney Disease Quality Outcomes Initiative. Clinical practice guidelines for nutrition in chronic renal failure. American Journal of Kidney Disease 2000; 35 (supplement) S40-S41.

VIII. Resources

American Association of Kidney Patients
3505 East Frontage Road
Suite 315
Tampa, FL 33607
Phone: 1-800-749-2257 or (813) 636-8100
Email: info@aakp.org
Internet: www.aakp.org

Life Options Rehabilitation Program
c/o Education Institute Inc.
414 D'Onofrio Drive
Suite 200
Madison, WI 53711-1074
Phone: 1-800-468-7777 or (608) 232-2333
Email: lifeoptions@medmed.com
Internet: www.lifeoptions.org
www.kidneyschool.org

National Kidney Foundation Inc.
30 East 33rd Street
New York, NY 10016
Phone: 1-800-622-9010 or (212) 889-2210
Email: info@kidney.org
Internet: www.kidney.org